A Bucket

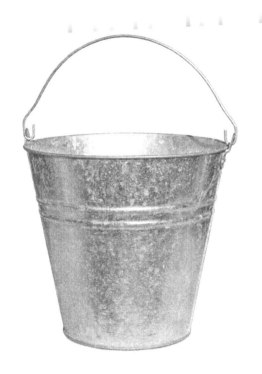

JAMES TOOMBS, MD

Disclaimer

The contents of this publication are intended to provide general information to a general public. The contents of this publication are no substitute for the medical diagnosis, advice or treatment from a licensed physician or other expert medical professional who personally examines you or your personal health information. All readers should seek personal consultation with and personal examination by a licensed physician or expert medical professional of their own choosing before commencing or adopting any exercise program, diet, or any other health-influencing practice for any general or specific health issue.

Author and publisher disclaim all responsibility for any liability, loss, or damage caused or alleged to be caused directly or indirectly as a consequence of the use, application or interpretation of the information in this publication.

ISBN: 0615764142
ISBN-13: 978-0615764146
Library of Congress Control Number: 2013932863
Pisacano Leadership Foundation, Lexington, KY

...bright graduates were hired, and their talent was continually recognized and rewarded. Work always ended early on Friday afternoons, but this day was special. After lunch, the staff gathered in the conference room. Promptly at half past one, the company's president—a familiar, cheerful icon—stepped up to the podium. A life-size cardboard cutout of the honoree stood to one side of the lectern. He paused a moment for conversations to wrap up, then asked the modest group, "Has it really been ten years? Jack, will you please join me?"

With a shiver of pride, Jack smiled and stepped up to shake hands with his boss. In this tight-knit company, anniversaries were milestones and always acknowledged. After a decade, Jack was still a relative newcomer, though clearly a rising star. He smiled again when he saw his wife, Jillian, and their daughter standing in the back. Jack felt a blush warm his face as the tribute began. Everyone on his team stepped forward to share a story.

After an hour of tales, cake, and punch, the president politely evaporated, his clear indication that the weekend could begin. Jack enjoyed a few more laughs and then gathered his family. He headed for the employee parking, still beaming.

"What will you do with that?" his wife asked when Jack entered the kitchen carrying the cutout under his arm.

He glanced down at his own face. "Not sure, but I can't throw him away just yet, can I? Do you have any ideas for dinner?" he asked with a grin.

———◦———

Sundaes at Sally's had followed lasagna at Luigi's, their Friday-night tradition. When they returned home, it was just past dark, and he was a little past full—stuffed, in fact. The girls headed upstairs to change into pajamas for movie night, another tradition. Jack stood in the kitchen, flipping through the day's mail. He glanced at the younger twin he'd left standing near the counter.

The picture had been taken on his first day at work. By his current appraisal, the hair was far too long, and the glasses frames were just a bit too clunky. On the other hand, the muscular chest virtually glowed through his white shirt. Jack nodded approvingly at this trim athlete and thought about high school. On a dare, he had joined the cross-country team with a friend and found he enjoyed running. He'd never been a standout runner—he had never finished higher than twelfth place. In college, he kept with it, running a few days every week. After a summer course in lifting, Jack also made daily use of the weight room in his dorm. These efforts were clearly visible in the cutout.

Setting the mail aside, he glanced up at the kitchen window. This reflection placed him virtually shoulder to shoulder with his younger self. His attention was now drawn to the figure beside the athlete. While the silhouette was similar, there were some obvious differences. The face was fuller, with the beginnings of a double chin. The shoulders now appeared to sag. Jack's eyes then came to rest on the roll just above his belt. It strained the buttons of his shirt, and Jack acknowledged aloud, "I ate too much tonight." Mentally committed to sit-ups in the morning, he climbed the stairs, smiling again.

Any thought of exercise had already vanished when Jack woke up Saturday morning to a singsong, "Daddy! Daddy!

iep, that was Daddy just out of college."

He was stunned by her next question.

"Why were you so skinny?"

Jillian's entrance rescued him from answering, but he spent more than a few minutes pondering his daughter's observation. After breakfast, he placed the cutout in the garage.

Sunday morning, one nagging thought roused Jack. From under a dusty pile of shoes, he retrieved the bathroom scale and approached it cautiously, wearing just his boxers. His step was gentle, but there was no fooling the scale. The needle swung broadly, resting just beyond two hundred. Quite loudly, he stated, "That can't be right," before he weighed himself two more times with the same results.

He quickly slid the scale back with his foot and grabbed a leather belt. Every belt hole showed some wear, but the final hole, stretched to an oval, confirmed what he already knew. "I've gotten fat," Jack said honestly and accurately.

Up until this very moment in his life, Jack had never worried about his weight. He had never paid any attention to it. He ate breakfast, lunch, and dinner—and, most days, several snacks too. He ate what he wanted. Until he surveyed himself next to the cutout, he was unaware, on any conscious level that his body had changed. He had no good plan how to get it back.

Jack's idea of weight loss was a high school wrestler dripping sweat while jogging in a plastic suit. Dieting? That was something his mother had tried occasionally, almost always with carrot sticks and baked fish.

At breakfast, Jillian knew something was wrong when Jack refused a second stack of waffles. "Not hungry?" she asked.

"Not pleased is more like it. I've put on thirty pounds since college—all right here," he said while shaking his belly for emphasis. "I don't know how I've gotten so heavy. I still eat exactly the same."

Acknowledging his concern, she responded, "Honey, we've both gained some weight. It just happens as you get older. We'll start watching a little closer, and it will come off."

Jack nodded slowly but still stewed inside as he took his plate to the sink. The rest of the day, he ate cautiously then rewarded himself with large slice of cake after dinner for his sacrifices.

———

A good night's sleep completely erased any worries. On Monday morning, Jack woke to the alarm and then showered and dressed in his normal routine. Breakfast with Jillian and Denise passed without a word about weight or dieting or cutouts or college. On the way to work, he dropped the convertible top and enjoyed the crisp morning air. At the coffee shop's drive-through, the barista knowingly queried, "The usual?"

Jack nodded. Minutes later, he arrived at his office.

Jacket off and sleeves rolled to the elbow, Jack sat, sipping latte and examining his anniversary plaque. Looking around the room, he considered where it should be hung. He set it aside and pulled a pile of papers from his inbox.

In the stack were a few party pictures, and Jack grinned as he flipped through them. Then he froze. Someone had captured a candid image of him with his arm around the cutout. "*Twins?*" was written in the margin. It was jest, of course, but struck a

chair. What's on your mind?"

Jack started slowly, but he ultimately confessed his underlying purpose. "I'm up about thirty pounds since college, and I'm not about to ask my wife about dieting. You lost a bunch of weight last year, and I'm wondering if you can point me in the right direction."

Sensing Jack's embarrassment, Aaron responded, "I did have the same struggle, much worse than thirty pounds. And, just like you, I tried dieting, but I was really without a clue. Through the grapevine, I'd heard the boss hired a part-time doctor, mostly for wellness. His name is Dr. Williams. You may know him; he gave the flu shots last winter. I ended up meeting with him several times, and since then it's been pretty easy to keep trim. The doc only works half a day a week, but you're in luck: it's Monday. He should be here this afternoon, from noon to five, I think."

———✦———

Back in his office, Jack added a small note to his calendar: "Dr. Williams - 1 p.m."

 Start Today!

ing to find Employee Health. It was right at quarter past one when he found the sign and pushed open the door. Jack discovered instantly that there was no waiting room. The smallish office was sparsely furnished with a desk and two chairs. At the desk was a balding, elderly gentleman hammering away furiously at the keyboard. He paused and looked up as the door opened fully.

"Dr. Williams?"

The man nodded affirmatively.

"I'm Jack Reynolds from purchasing. Do you have time to see me this afternoon? If you're busy, I can come back later."

Dr. Williams pushed his keyboard aside as he stood and offered his hand.

"Good to meet you, Jack. Now is perfect. Please, sit down and let me know how I can help you."

Without relaxing, Jack settled into the chair facing the desk. He couldn't help but notice the doctor's physique. Despite an aged face and white hair, the doctor appeared anything but frail. With some hesitation, Jack bore through the story of the cutout and his weight gain since college.

After a long pause, Dr. Williams commented, "Sounds pretty normal."

Jack's face posed the question, "What do you mean?" But before he could speak, Dr. Williams resumed.

"Consider our genetic heritage. One hundred thousand years ago, humans spent the day roving the forest looking for food. Berries, roots, nuts; they trapped squirrels and rabbits and even hunted deer occasionally. Every day was a quest—sometimes they feasted, other times they came up short. With no good methods to store food, they had to eat when food was available. Our ancestors developed an ability to accumulate fat; a buffer against the environment. A survival tool, not only for bad hunting days but winter too. You have those same survival genes. Where food is plentiful, it's natural for humans to pack on fat."

He waited to let Jack reflect and then resumed. "You said nothing has changed in how you eat since graduation. That's probably true and likely part of the issue. Before we jump into anything, let's take an inventory first. For the next week, all I want you to do is write down everything you consume—a complete food diary. Everything, even drinks and water, gets recorded. A simple entry: 'eggs, toast, and coffee for breakfast.' That's all I'm after."

Dr. Williams produced a small, blue, hardcover journal from a drawer and handed it across the desk. "Use this."

Jack opened it, discovering only lined pages, while Dr. Williams went on. "Let's meet again next week. Bring the diary back, and I'll go through it. Before you go, I'd like to get a few measurements."

The physician had Jack empty his pockets and kick off his shoes before stepping onto a scale. It was a traditional upright medical model, but, oddly, the numbers had been removed. That mattered little to the physician as he recorded Jack's weight and height without comment. The doctor then used a body tape to measure around Jack's neck and waist.

"Stay off your bathroom scale; we'll only use this one for now," Dr. Williams said while scratching a few notes on a clipboard.

Jack put his shoes back on and refilled his pockets. They both stood, and the doctor extended his hand. "Good to meet you, Jack. You'll do fine."

As he pulled open the door for Jack to leave, Dr Williams tapped the old

Once seated behind his desk, Jack dutifully recorded the sip of water he'd had on his walk back to his office and then resumed working.

Just before five, he shut off his computer and opened the journal. The afternoon's tally included two sodas and a bag of chips. He debated omitting the chocolate kisses he'd snagged from the receptionist. Grudgingly, he added them and then picked up his jacket to leave.

Aaron was waiting in the lobby and pointed to the journal as Jack walked up. His only remark was, "That's where it starts," as they walked to their cars.

Jack brought the journal to the dinner table. Denise explored the little book while he quizzed her about school. When she handed it back and began eating, he turned his attention to Jillian.

She listened attentively as, between bites of roast and potatoes, he detailed the short visit with Dr. Williams. After banana pudding, he quickly jotted down the meal and rose to help clean up.

The evening continued with some TV time and a game of Uno before Denise was toddled off to bed. Two hours and one bad movie later, Jack and Jillian headed upstairs for bed. He brought the journal to add his movie snack: dry cereal.

Jack logged the day's final entry and set the journal on the nightstand.

"You're really serious about this," Jillian finally asked, more comment than question.

With a yawn, Jack sighed, "Yes, but I'm not sure how this will help."

Jillian had a keen interest in Jack's newfound weight-loss goal. The frustrations with her figure began at puberty. Since then, her weight was quite variable, moving with monthly cycles and the season. Before Denise, growing curves were wrangled into submission with periodic dieting. In a few weeks, an uncomfortable eight would melt back to her usual six, and she could eat again. Now, six years after giving birth, her body still held tight to twenty of the thirty-five pounds she'd gained while pregnant. She had tried dieting several times, but the extra pounds seemed to be a permanent fixture.

While Jack brushed his teeth, Jillian rummaged through several drawers to find a notepad of her own. When she returned, Jack was propped up in bed with the remote, slowly scanning channels. She plopped onto the bed beside him. An hour later, she heard him snoring. She clicked off the TV and fell quickly asleep too.

 Know what you are eating.

 Start keeping a food diary.

Monday afternoon, he took a break from work and headed to Employee Health.

As before, Dr. Williams was clacking on the keyboard when Jack entered. A smile grew on the doctor's face when he rose to greet Jack. "Thanks for coming in today."

He accepted the journal and set it square on his desk. "I want to review your diary, but let's get your weight first."

In stocking feet, Jack stepped onto the scale and, again, the doctor made a note without any remark, and then both men sat. Jack picked up his shoes, and the doctor picked up the journal and leaned back in his chair.

Jack was more than a bit uncomfortable as the doctor slowly examined each page. He waited silently, scanning the small room with his eyes. They came to rest on a framed diploma perched on a short bookshelf. From the date, he quickly calculated the doctor was probably thirty years his senior. "Looks pretty healthy for sixty-five," he thought.

Dr. Williams snapped the diary closed, and Jack's attention snapped back as well. He was quite surprised with the doctor's appraisal. "You did a great job. I ask patients to keep food diaries because it brings some attention back to eating. Human recall is remarkably imperfect. If you ask a man what he had to eat on a particular day, on average, he'd miss about 40 percent of the calories. With a diary, it's down in black and white. And people start making changes when they're more aware."

"Your meal pattern—breakfast, lunch, and dinner—is very good; humans need to eat regularly. Starting the morning with breakfast jump-starts your metabolism. Skipping any meal can lead to a demanding hunger and overcompensation later in the day. I see you snack between meals—that's human nature and a good habit too. Our ancestors ate small amounts many times a day simply because that's how they encountered food.

"Berries didn't grow in lush rows but were scattered all through the forest. It was a very lucky hunter who found a patch big enough to fill him up. The human digestive system is well designed to handle small frequent meals. Eating just once or twice a day can spell huge trouble. These less frequent meals tend to be bigger. They overload the system and start a man down the road to diabetes."

Dr. Williams continued, "At our last visit, I said that 'survivors get fat.' The human weight-control system is skewed to gain. We all have an internal drive that pushes us to eat beyond satiety. When balanced against food scarcity, this makes perfect sense. In our ancestor's environment, hunting and gathering was a full-time job. They engaged in *active* overconsumption when food was plentiful. This built fat, which was their defense against the inevitable unsuccessful hunts and cold winters. Nowadays, food is everywhere in whatever variety or quantity we choose. Though our so-called hunts are always successful now and a man can have twenty pounds of fat packed onto his belly, the appetite still demands we eat. The result is chronic *passive* overconsumption, and we slide toward obesity. In 2012, more than 70 percent of adults in America are overweight or obese—or even worse. Instead of expected seasonal weight variations, slow progressive gain is now the normal human experience.

"Humans also tend to engage in *mindless* eating: munching away when the brain is otherwise distracted. Sometimes it's grabbing a bite of this or a handful of that as we pass through the office or kitchen. Other times, it's snacking away at a bag of chips while typing reports. If I'm not cautious, I can find myself halfway through a tub of popcorn thirty minutes into a movie. It

would you be surprised to hear you've lost two pounds?"

The astonishment was clear on Jack's face. He was about to ask how but didn't get the chance.

The doctor handed back Jack's journal. "You're on the right track. For the next week, continue the diary, but I would like you to add an element of quantity. On most prepackaged foods, there are nutritional facts somewhere on the box. Measure your serving, and then note the calories in your journal. For everything else, fresh vegetables or meat, just note the volume or weight: one cup of broccoli or six ounces of steak, for example. You'll need a food scale and some measuring cups. We need to get another measurement too."

The doctor retrieved a black, pager-sized device and passed it to Jack. "I'd also like you to wear this on your belt or waistband. Put it on as soon as you get up, and take it off just before bed. It will help me give you some additional direction, but more on that next week."

As both men stood, Jack clipped it over his left hip.

———

Back at his desk, Jack thumbed through his diary. He was happy to be down two pounds but curious how this was working.

In review, there were only two real changes he could point out: he had chosen a cone over his usual hot fudge concoction at Sally's and refused a second pork chop at Sunday dinner. He thought about how easy it was to eat in contrast to the struggles of his ancestors. The phone rang; he closed the book and plunged back into work.

On the way home, Jack stopped and purchased a small digital scale and plastic measuring cups. He brought them to the table when Jillian called him to dinner. Steak, green beans, and potatoes—Jillian watched him measure each one as he added them to his plate. Denise broke the silence.

"What are you doing, Daddy?"

He responded, "Just checking my food. Wanna try?"

He slid the scale in front of her and showed her how to work the buttons. For the rest of dinner, he and Denise took turns weighing food, and it became a game.

Later that evening, after Denise was already asleep, Jack and Jillian headed to the basement to watch a DVD. She noticed he brought only a bowl of cereal and not the whole box. She usually shared this movie snack with him. Jack endured the look of protest for ten seconds and then produced a paper cup from his pocket and scooped some up for her.

 Know how much you are eating.

 Add food weights and measures.

curiosity about the device on his belt was killing him. Dr. Williams retrieved both as Jack began emptying his pockets and untying his shoes.

After stepping off the scale, Jack sat, waiting silently as the doctor read through his diary. Five minutes and seven pages later, Dr. Williams scribbled a few notes and then set the book aside. Jacked hoped for some critique, but instead the doctor asked, "What did you learn when you started adding quantities to your diary?"

Jack hesitated before blurting out, "I'm eating too much."

"My wife was surprised the first night I brought the cups and scale to the dinner table and weighed everything. Now, she weighs her food too. It's a bit awkward, but we're using the measuring cups to serve food. Pretty messy for mashed potatoes, but at least the servings are consistent. My daughter thinks it's fun. One day, I'm hoping we can go back to spoons. I got the big shock when I started paying attention to food labels: one ounce of this or half a cup of that. I saw my usual helpings were always bigger than what was considered a serving, according to the packaging. A serving of ice cream is only half a cup, just enough for a taste. I'll snack on a small bag of chips, and that's considered two servings.

"I know I've cut back some. If I have seconds, it's just a little more, not another plate like I used to. Going out for lunch or, for that matter, eating anywhere but home is still a real problem, though. I can't measure anything, and I just have to guess."

With a frustrated sigh, Jack fell silent. As if on cue, Dr. Williams began.

"Everyone I've worked with has been surprised when they start measuring instead of guessing. This is how awareness brings change. Sounds like it's working for you. After a week or two, you'll have a recalibrated serving size. Then you can go back to the spoons—if your daughter will allow it."

Dr. Williams laughed and went on, "Have you ever eaten too much at Thanksgiving? Of course, everyone has. All that food and all those tastes—we can't help ourselves.

"When we eat, every area of the digestive system sends signals to the brain, describing the meal. There are also some stretch receptors in the stomach that call out 'whoa' when it's full. All these signals move pretty slowly, so it's easy to overshoot and overeat. Some of my patients use a few techniques—speed bumps, really—to slow eating and let the system work. They serve in courses: salad first, then the meal, and then dessert. Plates are prepared in the kitchen, not on the table, so that if you want more, you have to take a few extra steps. The goal is finishing well shy of uncomfortably full. When you're loading the dishwasher, you'll feel good, not stuffed.

"You're exactly right about eating outside the home. In general, people eat more at restaurants. Even when they provide calorie counts, fast-food outlets and restaurants are still ripe for overeating. The servings are usually huge, and I, like most people, feel guilty about wasting food. Before I even sit down, I have a plan, like ordering just an appetizer or salad. When I'm set on a full meal, I split it down the middle right off and take half home. Most days, however, I pack my own lunch. That way I know exactly what I'm getting.

"But enough about food. I'll bet you're curious about this," Dr. Williams said while picking up the device and opening it with a small tool.

"It's a pedometer, a simple counter of the steps you take. I

Dr. Williams then asked the loaded question: "Jack, how far do you think you walk every day?"

Jack thought about his daily travels, wandering through the house, the distance from the parking lot to the office, all the trips to the printer and fax room, walking to the mailbox, and shopping some evenings. "No more than five or six miles, I'd guess."

After typing a few numbers into his calculator, Dr. Williams remarked, "Would you believe slightly less than three miles? Of course, that's an estimate, but probably not off by more than one-fourth of a mile or so. Over the past seven days, you took a total of 42,714 steps, which is about 6,102 steps per day. Using your height to approximate your stride, I came up with 2.8 miles. I see the frown, but, Jack, you're in good company. The average American only takes about 6,600 steps per day.

"Even adding two thousand steps can make a real difference in your weight in the long run. That's about a mile per day. A two hundred-pound man burns about one hundred calories walking that extra mile. Since there are 3,500 calories in a pound of fat—I'm fudging the math a bit—if you walk an extra mile every day, you'll burn off a pound of fat every month. Again, small changes pay off big in the long-term."

Dr. Williams then passed Jack a different pedometer. This model opened like a clamshell to reveal the counter and controls.

Dr. Williams showed Jack how to work it and gave him instructions to record the numbers and reset the counter every night.

As Jack clipped it to his belt, the doctor asked, "Would you be surprised to hear you've lost another two pounds?"

Jack subtly hooked a thumb inside the waistband of his pants. He'd lost four pounds total. Were his pants loosening, or was this just his imagination?

The doctor stood and moved to the door as Jack picked up his diary. "Next week, I'd like you to bring your wife, but only if she's eager to accompany you. Weight is a family affair, and when you start making changes at home, she'll need to participate. But it does sound as if she's already interested in your program. Just in case, here's a pedometer for her too."

In bed that night, Jack gave Jillian all the details about the visit, including his weight loss. When he asked her to go with him the following week, she thought her "Yes!" sounded just a bit too eager. She blushed and continued, "I've not been happy with my body for the past few years. Really, it's been more like six—since Denise was born. The old diets just don't seem to work anymore. I'm kind of jealous that you're losing weight and not suffering like I used to."

Jillian told Jack she had started a food diary too. She was wondering where to pick up a pedometer when Jack handed the extra one to her. She thought she was starting to lose some weight already, but she couldn't find the scale to check.

"Jack, honey, where did you hide it?"

 Move the mark.

 Involve your family.

Recording everything had slowed her snacking considerably, and she'd lost four pounds so far.

After getting dressed, she checked her shape in the mirror. "Hmm."

Four pounds was just a fraction of what she wanted to lose; she could not see any change in her reflection yet. This program was taking longer than her usual crash diets. On the other hand, she wasn't suffering. In the closet, Jillian reached for her shoes and saw the blue dress. She touched the sleeve and remembered wearing it. It had been purchased specifically for her sorority's five-year reunion. Like everyone, she wanted to hear, "You haven't changed a bit."

In preparation, she had joined a local fitness club where a personal trainer helped her build a workout routine. Sweating in the gym three days a week was hard, but the results were amazing. She had even felt comfortable in a two-piece that summer—the first time since college.

Jillian ensured her diary was up to date then drove to meet Jack for lunch. She phoned him as she pulled into the parking lot.

"I'll be right down," he told her.

Jillian's car was idling in a visitor's space when he came out the building. Jack walked directly to her door instead of the passenger's side. He opened it just slightly.

"It's beautiful today. Would you like to walk?"

Jillian switched off the motor and reached for her purse. "This seems more and more like when we were dating," she thought as she stepped out of the car.

Last Friday, they split a dinner, for the first time since college. They'd also gone on an after-dinner walk twice. Denise had ridden her bicycle beside them the whole way.

Jack kissed her cheek. "I found this place last week. They have a few salads I think you'll like. Are your shoes OK for walking? It's about half a mile there and back."

———

Lunch complete, they strolled back to Jack's office. He picked up his diary and added the appetizer and salad they'd shared. Jillian's journal was already complete and tucked back into her purse. At Employee Health, Jack knocked before pushing the door open.

Dr. Williams moved from behind the desk to greet them both. Jack introduced Jillian. She offered her hand and noticed the doctor's calluses as they shook. It struck her as odd that a physician would have such rough hands. When Jack handed over his diary to the physician, she did the same. She watched Jack while he went through the usual routine of emptying pockets and removing shoes. She drew a deep breath when Jack stepped onto the scale, "Oh no!" she though. She exhaled, relieved, when the physician motioned her to sit.

After reading the scale, Dr. Williams entered a note and began as Jack retied his shoes. He turned his attention to Jillian. "Thank you for coming with Jack today. I'm happy to see you've kept a food diary. Are you wearing the pedometer too?"

She patted her hip and nodded.

"Jillian, we don't have a reference weight, so I won't ask you to weigh here. Do you have a good scale at home?"

She nodded again.

"Great. I strongly recommend tracking weight. It helps measure the effect of changes you're making while reinforcing success. Patients who self-monitor with a scale are much

on track."

The doctor picked up Jack's diary and began reading, pausing after every page to enter the daily step count into his calculator. "Jack, if my totals are correct, you took more than sixty thousand steps for the week. We'd set a daily goal of 8,000 steps, but on average, you took 8,321. You've added more than a mile a day. My question is how?"

Jack beamed. He had been walking extra every day to build his total. "I've done a few easy things, like parking on the far side of the lot and walking in the evenings with Jillian and Denise. When it's nice and I have the time, instead of driving to lunch, I'll go on foot."

Jillian was slightly nervous when Dr. William picked up her diary. He looked at her before opening it and politely asked, "May I?"

She answered simply: "Please do."

He started with her last entry and slowly paged backward, typing numbers into his calculator as he went. After a few minutes, he looked up. "I've totaled the past seven days, and your average is 9,881. For healthy adults, ten thousand steps a day is linked to some solid health benefits, and you're right on the mark. I'm guessing that you're about five feet, four inches tall."

He paused, then, hearing no correction, Dr. Williams continued with a few more strokes on his calculator. "So, that's right over four miles. Very good."

Hearing this reinforced Jillian's commitment to a morning walk after getting Denise off to school.

Dr. Williams went on. "I do have a concern about your meal pattern. Most days, it looks like you skip breakfast. Almost one-fourth of Americans do. I'd encourage you to have at least a little something in the morning. Long-term studies show breakfast eaters weigh less, and it seems to be related to the insulin response and fat storage. Humans wake after a ten-hour fast with bellies and bodies ready for a meal. The longer we wait before eating, the stronger the insulin response grows. This seems to prime the body for fat storage. A small bowl of cereal and a piece of fruit is adequate if you're not a breakfast person."

Dr. Williams closed her diary and handed it back. "You may also find you have more energy in the morning too."

Dr. Williams opened Jack's diary again. "Let's talk a little more about snacks. A few weeks back, I said they were a good habit. Humans are natural grazers, and a mid-morning snack will likely help prevent overeating at lunch. Studies show more frequent eating can also even out the body's insulin response to help prevent diabetes. Unfortunately, we usually choose snacks by convenience—whatever happens to be handy. More often than not, convenience spells sugar and fat. During the week, Jack, it looks like you always have a snack in the morning, then one or two in the afternoon. Your usual is a soda and a bag of chips or a cookie."

Jack squirmed a little in his chair while the doctor continued.

"Your current habits in both diet and exercise have been formed over the past ten years. Right now, they feel natural and comfortable to you. But these are the very same habits that helped you gain an *uncomfortable* thirty pounds. Over the past few visits, you started a diary and increased your walking. Over the next several weeks, you'll make even more changes.

"In short order, these actions will become more natural, and eventually your new routine. There is no miracle in play; it's

Jack quickly responded, "Bananas."

The doctor's face lit up. "Very good. The humble banana has potassium, which is good for your kidneys and bones; loads of fiber; and a fair amount of vitamin B6. No preparation required, just peel and eat. All that for only one hundred calories.

"For the rest of this week, try bringing a banana from home every day, and let some of the chips linger in the vending machine."

The doctor paused and returned Jack's diary. "Getting healthy is not about giving up all the foods you love. Have you ever tried the brownies that Maryann bakes? They're my favorite. I check the break room every Monday when I arrive. A whole one, however, is not part of my program."

Those brownies were beyond great; they were legendary. Jack had always wondered who could take only half, and now he knew. Point understood.

Dr. Williams stood and walked around the desk. "Jack, in total, I have your weight down six pounds over three weeks. That's remarkable but, with the efforts you've made, not at all unexpected. Let's meet again next week. Jillian, I appreciate you being here today. You're always welcome."

The couple left the office, and, as the door closed behind them, a lively conversation started about walking and shopping.

When they reached her car, Jillian agreed to pick up bananas and more cereal on her way home.

 Breakfast is essential.

 Improve snacking with intelligent trades.

... chocolate

... Jack pulled a plastic knife ...momentarily, and then cut one in half. ...on, he placed the smaller piece on a napkin and ... back to his office. Mission accomplished.

At his desk, Jack dutifully noted the morning snack and then paged back through his diary as he nibbled. Since the last visit with Dr. Williams, he'd replaced his afternoon potato chips with a banana. That trade, Jack figured, was saving him at least a hundred calories per day. Small changes, just like the doctor ordered. He lifted the final crumbs of his morning treat with a finger, crumbled the napkin, and returned to his computer.

Jillian had dropped Denise off at school, changed quickly, and then left for her morning walk. The big loop of the neighborhood was 2,614 steps. She had driven the route in her car last week, confirming it was just over a mile. She walked two laps most days, three if her schedule allowed. Listening to music or books on tape, the time passed easily. Nearly every day now, her step count was exceeding eleven thousand.

When Jillian returned home, she went upstairs, undressed for the shower, and weighed herself. No change from yesterday, but compared to last week, she was down a pound. While the water warmed, she checked her shape in the mirror again.

She'd lost five pounds total. "From where?" she questioned as she stepped into the shower.

That query faded instantly as the water hit her shoulders and she began planning the rest of the morning. "Lunch, today, will be a picnic."

Jillian repacked the basket after their meal and returned it to her car. Jack had been pleasantly surprised with her choice: chicken sandwiches under the pavilion on a perfect fall day.

At one o'clock, they promptly made their way to Dr. William's office. Jack knocked softly and then pushed open the door. For once, the doctor was not working at the computer but reading.

He set the magazine aside and stood to greet the couple. "Jack, it's good to see you. Jillian, thanks for coming in again."

Without prompting, they handed him their diaries. Their movements were so similar it appeared choreographed, and the doctor had to laugh. He motioned them both to sit, and Jack began untying his shoes.

Even before Jack stepped on the scale, he knew he had done well. He'd been tracking his weight at home and believed he had lost more than a pound since last Monday. Dr. Williams made a note silently, and Jack returned to his chair.

"This morning," the doctor began. "I found my brownie already cut and was curious. Who else in this office has a will of steel?"

Dr. Williams opened Jack's diary and read the last few entries. "So, it's you!" he said with mock surprise.

Jack just smiled. "By my records, you've lost another two pounds, for a total of eight pounds over four weeks. That's excellent!

"Eight pounds is almost 5 percent of your body weight. What have you noticed?"

Almost embarrassed by his success, Jack spoke softly, "I moved up a notch on my belt."

Jillian was surprised at the doctor's response. "That's excellent too. Percentage-wise, I'll bet you've lost as much as Jack, perhaps more. When shedding pounds, I've always thought spouses should avoid any pound-for-pound comparison. Men have a few advantages with weight loss. Let's say a man and his wife both cut their food intake by 20 percent. The husband drops his daily calories from 2,500 per day to 2,000. That deficit of 500 calories totals 3,500 for the week, equivalent to a pound of fat. His wife weighs substantially less, and, of course, she eats proportionately less. When she cuts her calories by 20 percent, perhaps by 350 calories per day, it takes ten days to lose the same pound of fat. Seven days versus ten days. Men also burn more calories exercising, but only because it takes more energy to move more weight. A 200-pound man burns more than one hundred calories walking a mile; his 135-pound wife burns just seventy-four. She'll have to walk almost fifty miles to burn off a pound, while he's down a pound after only thirty-five.

"You can't tell your body where to lose weight. How humans add fat is strictly genetic and different for men and women. Weight loss follows the same pattern, but in reverse. Last pound on is the first off is how I describe it. Men tend to carry a high percentage of their body fat right in the belly. With even the very first pounds of weight loss, they might notice, like Jack, a change in their pants size. Women don't gain so specifically. When they add fat, some goes to the belly, but more goes to the thighs, buttocks, and breasts. With weight loss, it's slowly drained from all these separate areas. My poor analogy is this: trim a layer off an onion, and you might not be able to tell it's any smaller. That's the typical female pattern. Now when you take a slice from an onion, even a thin one, anyone can spot the difference. There's the man's advantage. Have patience. This is a lifetime plan, and I'd say you both are right on target."

Jillian's relief in Dr. Williams' explanation was apparent as she relaxed in her chair.

The doctor eased back too and began reviewing diaries. He made several notes and then looked up. "It's tough to study humans thoroughly. Medical experiments necessarily have a very narrow focus. On the other hand, if we ask a large number of people about habits and note their medical conditions, we're able to form a general opinion about what's healthy. That's how scientists developed the ten-thousand-steps-per-day recommendation. Big population studies showed, again and again, the healthiest adults move more. Another habit of the healthiest adults is eating foods that have low calorie density and high nutrient content, such as fruits and vegetables.

"Years ago, a government agency began promoting the 5-A-Day plan. For adults, the very basic advice was to eat at least five servings of fruits and vegetables every day. It was easy to remember and easy to track. Their recommendation makes good sense medically and translates into better health long-term. Regarding weight, the high water and fiber content of fruits and vegetables make them filling—ideal for decreasing your overall calorie intake. The idea is not simply tacking on extra fruits and vegetables but using them to reduce or replace high-calorie items, like having a banana instead of chips."

Jack nodded slowly and realized, while the doctor appeared laid-back, he paid close attention to the details—their details.

Dr. Williams sat upright and faced the couple. "I've done a quick tally for both of you, following only two rules: fruit juices count toward your total. Potatoes, in any form, don't. By my count, Jillian, you had twenty-four fruit and vegetable servings last week, which ...

... apple slices—ours doesn't. I'd be tempted to grab the other half of the brownie or a package of cookies if I didn't have these."

The doctor reached into a desk drawer and produced a plastic bag full of blackberries.

"Part of the issue with Americans is that we're busy, and we eat what's available—whether at home, the office, or on the road. Having immediate access to fruits and vegetables clearly improves the chances of intake. I wish I'd known this when my children lived at home. Parental modeling, along with availability, helps kids establish a pattern of healthy eating. They cannot be persuaded or goaded or forced into eating right, but you can count on hunger. It always trumps preferences. When fruits are available and chips and candies aren't, guess what gets eaten? Your daughter has many more years before she leaves for college. That gives you time to influence her behaviors through modeling and access."

Dr. Williams let that idea settle for a moment.

"When I started paying careful attention to my health, I was blessed to have my wife's attention too. There were several months of subtle changes. Covertly, potato chips began disappearing from the pantry, and then, on our counter, a fruit bowl appeared. She made a point to add something colorful at every meal. While I never became a fan of the breakfast salad, a bowl of banana and orange slices suited me fine. I can even tolerate raw vegetables if she includes a little hummus for dipping. Slowly, this novel way of eating just became my normal.

"Jack, your afternoon banana is a big step. At first, it might seem impossible to trade chocolate-covered almonds for an apple, but you're looking at a man who gave up brownies for berries six days a week."

He handed the diaries back and stood. "Next Monday?"

Jillian went home and took inventory. In their pantry, she counted a half dozen different brands of chips. The plastic bowl they used to hand out Halloween candy was almost half full of bite-size chocolates. Vegetables, fruit cups, beans, and cereals were scattered throughout the shelves. "Let's rearrange this."

For the next hour, Jillian sorted, sifted, and finally separated their food into two groups. Stowed on the left side of the shelves were items they would use but not replace. The right side of the shelves held their healthy choices. Jillian planned to grow this, starting today.

Jillian grabbed her keys and then headed to the grocery store. She picked up Denise on the way home, carried in groceries, and began unloading. The youngster pulled a red and yellow fruit from one bag.

"That's a mango!" Denise declared. "We had one at Mary's house last Saturday. They're good."

Jillian smiled and thought, "This might not be so hard."

 You cannot tell your body where to lose fat.

 Five fruits and vegetables every day.

— and the fall colors were beautiful. She trekked three neighborhood loops and a little more just to finish her audio book. Afterwards, in the kitchen, Jillian opened her diary to add the apple she'd just bitten, her new late-morning snack. She quickly totaled fruits and vegetables for the past week. "Thirty-six so far," she said aloud.

She looked at the emerging pattern. Fruit with breakfast. Fruit for snacks. Salad, vegetable, or both with lunch and dinner. Overall, adjusting to 5 A Day was much easier than she'd expected. Jack was following it religiously and picked at least two items from the fruit bowl daily. With a little gentle coaching, Denise was changing her habits too. Getting started required combining fruit with old favorites: apple slices with yogurt or berries with ice cream.

"In time," she thought, "we'll simplify to plain fruit."

Jillian had already quit buying fruit bars and now bought only fresh fruit. Rather than a salad, Denise enjoyed crisp spinach leaves with her favorite dressing as a dipping sauce.

Jillian checked her watch and realized she'd have to hustle to make her noon lunch date with Jack. Upstairs, she stepped onto the scale without the usual dread. She had been weighing daily but recording only on Mondays.

No surprise, another pound was gone. The consistent trend down was giving her confidence in Dr. William's program. "And I'm not even starving."

After her shower, she stood wrapped in a towel and wondering, "What should I wear?"

In the closet, gazing at her wardrobe, the question changed to, "What could I wear?"

For the past year, she had avoided buying new clothes because it seemed like surrender to her current post-baby size. Unfortunately, it left her with far fewer choices. The blue dress was still off limits, but, down six pounds, last fall's slacks might just be possible. Jillian pulled a pair off the hanger, took a deep breath, and stepped into them.

Jack closed the file, slid back in his chair, and checked the clock. It was almost time for lunch with Jillian. He opened his diary, ensuring it was complete. An orange on Monday morning was an odd entry. For the first time in years, he'd passed right by the brownies.

"Half a brownie is good, but fruit is better. I wonder if he'll comment?"

Jack had come to enjoy the brief Monday meetings with Dr. Williams. What he enjoyed more was success. Jack believed he was down an honest ten pounds. A faint stomach growl prompted Jack to glance at the clock again.

He scooped up his diary, grabbed his jacket, and headed for the stairs. Jillian was just pulling onto the lot, so he walked to her car.

She stepped out, closed the door, and took one slow spin. "Notice anything different?" she asked in her best Mae West voice and with a broad smile.

"I believe those are new pants," Jack responded.

"No, honey, they're *old* pants." Impossibly, the smile grew even bigger.

———

, , ---- ... .. physician, I've come to understand that traditional diets, in any form—low-fat, low-carbohydrate, low-calorie—don't work. Sure, cutting calories to five hundred a day will drop pounds off anyone…for a while. But these diets create an environment of restraint, and the body will rebel. At some point, human nature seizes control, and most everyone resumes eating in the pattern that added pounds to begin with. Diets try to defeat human systems that are a million years old. Why not work with them?

"By trading away some high-calorie–dense foods and eating regularly throughout the day, we actually engage the normal human system. We still have the taste buds of hunter-gatherers, and, consistent with those survival instincts, we choose energy-dense foods, like meat. Even so, weight or volume, rather than energy content, is one of the most important determinants of meal size. In human studies, researchers can manipulate the calorie content of food items without changing the weight or volume. People tend to eat the same amounts, regardless. Even in time, the stomach doesn't learn energy content, nor do participants compensate for the different energy densities. Simply put, looking at the stomach as a scale, meat or mangoes, it all counts the same, and the meal is over when the stomach says full. Adding fruits and vegetables lowers energy density but involves little sacrifice. Does it work for weight loss? Sure does. And it's sustainable."

Jack turned slightly to his wife and said, "She gets the groceries and should get all the credit."

Jillian only blushed.

The doctor picked up both diaries. "I saw you've almost stopped eating potatoes completely. Overall, I think that's very good, but I should explain a little further. At last visit, I said that potatoes don't count as vegetables. Most of my patients will reflexively drop them from the menu. I've got nothing against spuds. The average medium potato has some heft— about six ounces—mostly carbohydrates, but a little protein too. In the natural form, they're low in fat and high in vitamin C. It's in the preparation or decoration that Americans ruin potatoes. They appear on our plates fried or drenched in cheese, butter, and sour cream. Suddenly, 150 calories of good nutrition jumps to 450 from added fat. If you keep potatoes in your diet, baked and seasoned is just fine. That brings me directly to another point.

"Several years ago, I read a study about the habits of some health professionals. A large group was tracked for two decades, and, every four years, the researchers asked them detailed questions about diet and activity. They also asked about weight. When they finally fed everything into a computer, several things popped right out. The first being that most people gained weight over twenty years. Fair enough, and not totally unexpected. When they looked closely at eating habits, the participants who gained the most weight regularly included three items in their diet: fries, chips, and soda."

When the doctor paused, Jack slumped slightly and began some mental calculations. He knew he'd be good on the first two, but the last was a real problem. Soda in the house was pretty rare, but he always drank two at his desk, and, maybe one or two with lunch. Before he could reach a total, the doctor resumed.

"It was easy for me to understand fries and chips, both have a high energy density, and they delight human taste buds. Fat and salt were rare treats in the caveman's diet. I had to dig a little deeper on soda, and it probably comes right down to habit. We like the sweet taste and it' [illegible] y, we don't. I could drink two liters on a hot summer day without ever feeling full. That's eight hundred calories, a whole meal.

"The liquid and simple sugars of soda don't require much digestion. They get absorbed quickly and skip our innate counters, so we don't even recognize the calories. That brings me around to the real issue. Other than breast milk in infancy, humans really aren't geared for drinking anything with calories. Our ancestors probably drank only water, and that's the best choice for modern humans too. Unless you're specifically having a fruit smoothie as a meal replacement, you're unknowingly adding calories and weight with liquid calories—whether in sodas, sweet tea, lattes, or milkshakes. I still like soda, but I've changed to limit myself to only one per day. There is some thought that the empty sweetness triggers our appetite, but diet soda drinkers don't add the pounds. Tea is another good choice and may have some cancer-preventing properties from the antioxidants. Just stay light on the sugar or use a natural sweetener.

"The biggest change I made years ago was keeping water handy. The only fountains in this building are located between the restrooms. That's too far to walk when you want just a sip. We do have a faucet and ice in the break room. Bottled is another fair option."

For the first time, Jillian noticed the doctor's water tumbler next to his monitor. As if reading her mind, he reached for it, took a drink, and went on. "Again, kids require some coaching. Our granddaughter just turned seven. Her parents have done a good job avoiding soda, and she is fine with milk or water at meals. Their one exception is 100 percent juice at breakfast. That does count as a fruit, as you know.

"Any questions today?"

His pause was met with silence. "No? By the way, Jack, you're down another two pounds. Ten total, in case you've lost count."

Before picking up Denise, Jillian made another trip to the grocery store. They were almost out of soda at home—the perfect time to switch. She looked up and down the rows, finally settling on their favorite brand in a zero-calorie variety. "I hope Jack will try this."

She also put a case of bottled water in the cart.

That evening, setting the table for dinner, Jillian casually asked Denise, "Did you want milk or water tonight?"

"Can I have both?" was the youngster's reply.

 The stomach is a simple scale.

 Limit beverages with calories.

...mochas, lattes, cappuccinos, and macchiatos. Sweet, steaming, and delicious. In ten years, he had tried them all.

After last week's visit with Dr. Williams, he decided to trade the froufrou versions for the shop's regular coffee. This lasted two days. When he dropped the fluff and calories, the stop seemed too pricey. Jack certainly wasn't a penny-pincher, but he couldn't see spending $2.25 for something offered free at work.

One night, Jack lamented the decision to Jillian. The next day, she found a big coffee mug and presented it to him with a bow. As he was filling it now, Jack's thoughts were drifting.

Jack's Monday morning was committed to a sales-team meeting. He had skipped breakfast to be at work early and make one final pass through his presentation slides. They were scheduled to end at noon. He hoped they would; his stomach was already growling.

The meeting did end a few minutes early. Jack glanced at his watch as he walked back to his office. There was just enough time to drop off his notes and grab his jacket. He trotted down the stairs and into the parking lot.

Jillian was just pulling in. He waved her up and leaned down to the open window. "I found a new place for lunch. It's not far, but let's drive today. I'm about to collapse."

She unlocked the doors, and he rounded the car and plopped into the passenger seat. The restaurant was a quick four minutes away. Despite a good lunch crowd, they were seated immediately. Jack munched on some chips while reviewing the menu. Instead of sharing a meal and salad today, he proposed they order separately. When the food arrived, Jillian asked for a to-go container and split her meal in half. Jack bore through his sandwich like a man possessed. When it was gone, he sat back to sip his tea.

"Better now?" Jillian asked teasingly.

Jack grunted, "Yep," and pulled out his diary.

Jillian stepped into Employee Health and presented Dr. Williams her diary. Jack trailed a few feet behind his wife.

"You look miserable," Dr. Williams said as they shook hands.

Jack quickly sat down, slid off his shoes, and related the morning's events. "I ate too much," he summarized succinctly.

He sighed when the doctor motioned him to the scale. After weighing in, Jack meekly returned to his chair.

"That one meal won't destroy your progress, but it does show how quickly the body adapts. I'll bet you've eaten a comparable sandwich many times this year without even flinching. More recently, however, you've changed how you eat. A small meal flanked by two snacks has replaced that big lunch. Your stomach has shrunk. It's a muscle and adjusts fairly quickly to meal size. Given smaller servings, in just a few weeks, the stomach capacity might shrink by a third. What you ate today was probably no more than what you ate six weeks ago. With your new eating plan, that old-sized meal put you well over full.

"Hunger was working against you too. When a man wakes up, he's already been fasting for twelve hours or so, and his body is ready for a meal. Skipping breakfast and your morning snack amplified the urge to eat. Hunger is the perfect spice. It practically commands humans to overeat when food suddenly becomes available. That's one of our earliest survival tools. It was essential when food was scarce but is essentially useless now.

And that's exactly why conventional dieting doesn't work. Diets impose restrictions, which activates our protective instincts and creates what I call *the hungry brain*. When the restrictions are lifted at the end of four, eight, or twelve weeks, we bounce right back to our pre-diet weight.

, ... On average, they lose a pound every three days. Over the eight weeks, a typical ranger candidate drops 12 percent of their body weight and burns off half their body fat. They start pretty lean and get even leaner. Some drop to as low as 5 percent fat, becoming emaciated. But after the training is over, they don't stay thin. In a few weeks, their weight rebounds and then climbs even higher than their entry weight, nearly twelve pounds higher. This recovery weight is virtually 100 percent fat. Three months after graduation, their body fat has ballooned to 21 percent. Jack, you've lost twelve pounds in six weeks, a pace only a little slower than the rangers. Other than today, I haven't heard you mention hunger. Why not?"

Jack's discomfort was gradually easing, as was his worry that he'd botched the program. But, he was stumped by the doctor's question. For a few awkward moments, there was only silence in the small office, and then Jack began to voice his thoughts. "I'm not hungry because I'm eating all the time. And, it's a ton of food. I go through my diary almost every night. Our meals are a whole lot better than just a few weeks ago. We're having fruit with breakfast, a vegetable or salad with lunch, and, almost always, two vegetables with dinner. At work, before I'm even thinking about it, I'll be in the break room washing my apple or peeling an orange. It seems I don't go but an hour or two before I'm eating again. Except for today, there's really never been a chance to get too hungry."

The doctor smiled broadly. "I'll give you an A for that answer."

He spent the next few minutes paging through their diaries and then swiveled his chair a bit to include Jillian. "I'm very impressed with the changes you've made. A caloric deficit is essential for weight loss, but it has to be created without waking the hungry brain. You've both been doing exactly that by adding more fruits and vegetables. Every day, I see at least five servings. And some days six or even seven. It's a higher volume of food with a much lower density of calories. Filling the belly soothes the brain, and hunger sleeps. In the standard diet, what gets you to goal isn't what keeps you at goal. Diets end, and weight rebounds. The eating pattern you've had for the past few weeks is one you can maintain forever; there's no three-month end point. And it doesn't have to be so rigid that you cannot have a cookie, or chocolate almonds, or even a big meal here and there."

The couple nodded in unison.

"I'd guess eating so frequently mimics grazing, but, for modern humans, it's more than that. We spend the bulk of our days just like this—sedentary: sitting and thinking. Sometimes with a pad of paper, other times hacking away at our computers. Cognitive work exerts a subtle pressure on appetite. A brain at work, calculating and coordinating, requires some extra calories. It runs solely on glucose and pulls what it needs directly from the blood stream. Sensing the slight drop in blood sugar, appetite switches on, and we start thinking about food. My solution, just like yours, is premeditated eating. It's become a firm habit to take bananas and berries to work so that I can avoid large lunches and visits to the vending room.

"While I eat frequently at work, sometimes I'm not entirely sure it's due to hunger. Food, in a historic context, was related to survival—the pure physical need for calories. In the modern context, food has a number of other roles, including comfort and reward, or a perceived want or need for calories. Planned, healthy eating is an effective strategy to help tame appetite, regardless of the origin. In my mind, that begs the question, what if we addressed the origin? In general, sedentary activities, like cognitive work and watch...

...rejuvenating the body's systems. Adults need seven or more hours a night, though most get far less. The key factor for weight control relates to cortisol, the stress hormone. A small amount of cortisol is released constantly. Much more is released during any perceived threat, boosting vigilance and preparing the body for action, the familiar fight or flight response. After the threat, cortisol helps the body recover by increasing appetite to replace fats and carbohydrates that were burned. During sleep, the release of cortisol is inhibited and levels decrease. Less sleep means more circulating cortisol, and that exerts another subtle pressure on the appetite. The effect of getting just four, five, or six hours of sleep might be too small to measure in a food diary, but not on the scale. The constant craving from cortisol inevitably leads to weight creep; twenty extra calories a day can add two pounds every year.

"I picture a caveman getting up at dawn and heading to bed near dusk, entrained with the environment. Even in the summer, that amounts to eight hours of sleep. Winters allowed much more. But who knows how much cavemen actually slept? What we do know is that, over the past one hundred years, human sleep patterns have changed dramatically: we sleep far less than we need. I blame it on the bulb. Humans still entrain with the environment, and light, in most any form, keeps us awake. With the invention of electric lighting, we can now stay busy after dark. I understand factories can manipulate lighting to help keep night-shift workers alert. But it's not just bright lights that affect sleep. Even television and computer screens mimic sunlight, increase alertness, and delay the onset of sleep. When I ask about sleep habits, some patients tell me they watch TV because they're not sleepy. I wonder if they're not sleepy because they're watching TV.

"From studying large groups, researchers determined that people with the best health get seven to nine hours of sleep. For most people, an alarm clock truncates the sleep window, regardless of the light outside. For that reason, sleep duration usually hinges on bedtime. All sorts of activities will push this back, so I'll have patients set a goal bedtime. It's simple: take your usual wake-up time, then subtract eight hours. That's bedtime, with lights out. Completely out. No TV, or laptops, or readers in bed.

"For the next week, I'd like you both to pay closer attention to sleeping habits, and consider the changes you'd have to make to target eight hours. I'd also have you survey your bedroom, thinking about the caveman and his dark sleeping environment."

The doctor passed back their diaries. "Jack, you're looking better. I think you'll survive."

That evening, Jack thought about sleep routines as he helped Denise to bed. Pajamas, flossing, brushing, potty, stories, prayers, hugs, kisses, and "good nights."

In just a few minutes, she was already softly snoring. He left her bedroom and went to his own. With the lights off, he sat on the bed and let his eyes adjust. Jillian pushed open the door slightly and whispered. "Jack?"

He stood and guided her to the edge of the bed. "Just wait."

In moments, the room seemed to brighten. Streetlights streamed in through their curtains. Green glowed from the cable box, computer, and television. The red rays from their smoke detector and alarm clocks cut across the bedroom. Jillian softly whispered, "This is no cave."

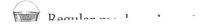 Regular

_____ ___ ____ upright. For the past few days, he and Jillian had made it to bed by half past ten—doctor's orders. While this was only marginally earlier than their previous routine, in sharp contrast, however, the TV remained off, and the reader was tucked away. They'd also made progress in building the cave by removing the night-light and a few glowing electronics and then adding window shades. "Not quite eight hours, but better," Jack thought as he turned on the lights.

"Maybe next week, we'll shoot for ten."

He heard his wife stirring behind him. Jillian yawned and said, "Good morning, honey," as she stood and slipped on her robe.

They exchanged a perfunctory morning kiss, and she headed downstairs. Jack finished his morning routine right on time to wake Denise for breakfast together. He opened her door, allowing the hallway light to spill in. "Time to wake up, Little Tiger."

———•———

With her family safely off to work and school, Jillian went out walking. She was consistently completing three laps each day, just over three miles. It took nearly an hour, but books on tape made the time quite tolerable. After her shower, she weighed before getting dressed.

She couldn't help but smile. The pounds were still evaporating—ten gone over the past seven weeks. She could look in the mirror and spot the differences. Her closet was filling up again; she'd added even more slacks and dresses from the spare bedroom. Jillian pulled the blue dress out and laid it across the bed. She placed her hands on her hips, comparing their width to the shape of the dress. "Tempting, but still off limits. Ten more to go, and then I'll try you on."

She checked the clock. There was still more than enough time to run her errands and meet Jack by noon.

———◦———

Over the past five weeks, Jack and Jillian had fallen into a comfortable Monday routine: lunch and then Dr. Williams. Today was perfect for outdoor dining, so they shared a large salad on the café's patio. Jack looked at Jillian on the walk back to the office. He patted his belly and said, "Much better this week."

At Employee Health, Jack knocked politely as they entered. They'd found him at the desk on other visits, but, today, Dr. Williams was fishing through the file cabinet. The doctor half turned to them and said, "Give me just a moment," before turning back to his search.

Jack and Jillian sat and placed their diaries on his desk. Jack unlaced his shoes, waiting and watching. A short minute passed. "Found you," the doctor whispered.

He placed a folder next to his computer and picked up Jack's chart. With a small wave, he motioned Jack to the scale.

As Jack returned to his chair after being weighed, the doctor began, "Weight gain. Weight loss. Either way, it boils down to a mismatch between caloric intake and expenditure. In our environment, there are so many cues to eat and ready access to all sorts of food. No wonder we usually gain. For the past seven weeks, Jack, you've been weighing, watching, recording, and losing steadily. Your progress has been exceptional so far, but…"

The doctor's voice trailed off momentarily, and Jack perked his ears. "This is the first ~~~~ ~~~~ ~~~~ ~~~~

~~~~~~gy. After losing thirteen pounds, your basic caloric needs probably dropped eighty to a hundred calories a day. Walking and moving take less energy too. I'm fairly certain there's some conservation; overall metabolism may slow somewhat. This helps preserve remaining fat—not your goal but historically necessary for survival. The body also has a sense of its set point and, perhaps, subtly encourages you to eat more. When intake matches expenditures again, you're at a plateau. I'd planned to talk about this today anyway, but now the timing is absolutely perfect."

The doctor opened the manila folder and extracted two, faded, black-and-white photographs. "Tell me, please, what in the world do these two men have in common?"

Jillian reached out and held the images so they both could see. She stifled a gasp. The print in her left hand showed a man with a towel wrapped double around his waist standing against a stark white background. His face was gaunt, and each rib was clearly defined; she could count every one. Jillian was sure her hand could close around his bicep. The second picture was a man cast against the same white background. He was clad in a towel tucked firmly underneath the drape of his enormous belly. His chest was a barrel; his arms thick as thighs. Jillian considered for a moment that it might be the same man, but the facial features and hairline were clearly different. She looked to Jack, then back to the doctor. She softly offered, "A prisoner and his guard?" as she laid the pictures back on the desk.

"Jillian, had I only seen their pictures, I would have guessed exactly the same, but I knew their story. They're actually friends—Olympic athletes on the same team."

Jillian was astonished and retrieved the pictures. As she scrutinized the photos more closely, the doctor leaned forward and tapped on one. "The young man here is a marathoner, and his comrade is a power lifter. Both were exceptional athletes in their events and won medals. A silver for the runner. A bronze for the lifter. This brings me squarely to the point: the body is exceptionally responsive to inputs and sculpted by applied forces. In long-distance running, there is a significant penalty for weight. With intense training and high mileage, fat diminishes, and even bones thin. Of course, when the demand is pure power, muscle recovery and growth both depend on food. And there's little penalty for a belly.

"These athletes are at the ends of the spectrum, but the same rules apply to ordinary people. The ideal body depends on what you do: with sedentary work, there are few demands physically, and virtually no penalties for excess weight. The most challenging task the common American worker faces is climbing one flight of stairs. It doesn't take much strength to operate a keyboard, and if that's all you do, muscles will slowly evaporate. Weight will continue creeping up with even the slightest excess of calories. After a few years, you'll have a body perfectly suited for office work."

The doctor retrieved both diaries, leafed through the pages, and placed a marker in each.

"In the first weeks of this program, you both changed eating habits, cutting calories significantly, and weight began falling off. Then you added more activity. For both of you, these changes to intake and activity are converging to produce your ideal body.

Jack, you've placed a primary focus on cutting calories. From today's weight, I imagine your trajectory is slowing, and you'll probably settle gently right at 180 pounds. That's an impressive 10 percent weight loss.

"Jill, you've made signif

…, and good sleep. Of course, keep moving too."

The doctor hesitated and then handed back their diaries. Jack pulled back his feet and readied to leave but noticed that Jillian was holding fast, as if she had a thought or question. The doctor was not moving either. Jack relaxed in his chair, and for a moment there was only silence.

"When individuals seek me out, I know they're seriously considering change. More often than not, weight is their primary concern. It's physically obvious and easily measurable. Over a few weeks, a few critical lifestyle modifications can induce a significant loss. You've both demonstrated this. Once we address that concern, a few patients are completely content and, for them, the official program is over. But there is a reason we call this Employee *Health*, not Employee *Weight*. If you'd like to make changes beyond a lighter weight, then I'll see you next week."

The doctor stood and extended his hand to both of them. "Thank you."

That night, Jack retrieved his cardboard double from the garage and brought it to the bedroom. Again, he stood shoulder to shoulder with it in front of a mirror. His body had changed over the past seven weeks. In some respects, he could see the movement toward his old shape, especially the belly. Another 7 pounds, if the doctor's 180-pound prediction was correct, would flatten it further. His shoulders were another story. "I'll never get those back by losing more weight," he conceded.

Jillian was brushing her teeth and watched Jack place the cut-out in their closet. Though he felt he knew the answer already he asked: "What are you doing next Monday?"

 The ideal body depends on what you do.

 Health is not just weight.

pounds and enough inches off his waist to merit new pants. He'd paid scrupulously strict attention to his diet for the past seven days. Even so, his weight was down only a pound, the second week in a row. "The doctor's forecast is probably right," he thought as he dressed for work.

———⚬———

Twenty minutes later, with his daughter in tow, Jack joined Jillian in the kitchen. While the youngster distributed forks and spoons, Jack sat with his coffee and watched his wife at the stove. She was already in her walking shorts, the tone in her calves emerging as she shifted from foot to foot. She turned with the skillet and caught Jack staring. He blushed and snapped his attention back to his empty plate. As she spooned scrambled eggs, Jillian spoke softly, "Honey, we only serve breakfast this time of the day."

———⚬———

Eager for a revelation, the couple finished a quick lunch and arrived at Employee Health promptly at one that afternoon. As they entered, Dr. Williams looked up from his magazine, swallowing the last bite of lunch with a sip from his thermos.

As Jack slipped off his shoes, Jillian slid their diaries onto the desk. The doctor folded his lunch bag and dropped it into a drawer. He stood, as did Jack, and they approached the scale together. The doctor jotted a note and returned to his chair.

"Jack, you're still moving in the right direction and down another pound, just like last week. Again, I believe you're moving toward a plateau."

Jack reclaimed his shoes while the doctor scanned their diaries.

"In helping patients move toward better health," the doctor began, "I've always started with weight loss first. Modest lifestyle modifications produce measurable changes, and that's very motivating for patients. A proper weight is clearly important but only one element of health. Though many patients are content with a purely lighter form, I understand you both want more. It's time we talked about *the bucket of life*."

Jack shot a confused look to Jillian, who reflected it right back. They turned simultaneously toward Dr. Williams.

"That facial expression appears every time I introduce the concept, so, let me spill the details.

"I was in the army for the first part of my medical career. The military has a crystal clear need for soldiers, even physicians, to be ready for overseas deployments. It's more than looking fit; they have to prove it. Every six months, soldiers have to meet weight standards. They also have to pass a physical fitness test that includes push-ups, sit-ups, and a timed run. They get some assistance, as physical training is built into the workday. For the most part, troops stay in good shape. The army's system of carrots and sticks brings the rest squarely into line. Overweight? Then no promotions.

"Failing the fitness test earns remedial workouts in the early mornings. Multiple failures might even bring discharge. Health was just part of the army's climate, and, when I retired at age fifty, mine was solid.

"I imagine the caveman's philosophy would be: eat when you can, move when you have to. Humans are quite efficient in building fat, and we naturally conserve energy. These are genetic traits that, only two hundred years ago, were essential for survival. After

he said.

"My wake-up call came one Sunday afternoon while working in the yard. It started with a little chest pressure, then a sharpness moved into my left arm. I dropped the shovel and went inside for a glass of water. My wife noted the pallor of my skin and that I was breathing rapidly, and, against my protests, she dialed 9-1-1. My color had returned by the time the ambulance arrived ten minutes later. When we got to the emergency room, I was feeling normal again and just wanted to go back to the yard. My wife prevailed, and I stayed, virtually chained to a hospital bed while they ran all the tests. Lying there, waiting for results, I saw the reflection in a wall mirror of a man beached on a hospital bed: an oxygen tube stuck in his nose and EKG leads tangled on his bare chest and big white belly. Up to that very moment, I still considered myself a soldier and still in good shape.

"The doctor was professional but pretty gruff. I don't recall much of what he said, except, 'Just a warning this time.' That last part, 'this time,' echoed in my head over and over. He said something else that caught me off guard: 'If you don't protect *the bucket*, you're going to kick it, sooner rather than later.'

"He ordered me to follow up with my primary care physician. I knew that was going to be a problem. Except the one in the mirror, I hadn't seen a doctor in five years.

"Finally, I was released, and I sulked home with my wife. I understood that, half the time, the very first sign of heart trouble in men is sudden death. I was beyond fifty, far overweight, and out of shape; perhaps I'd stopped working just in time. The shovel stayed in the yard where I left it.

"That night was pretty sleepless; I woke up committed to change, but I wasn't quite sure how. It was Monday, and there were already patients on my schedule. Later that day, I saw a physician, a friend of mine, who drew even more blood and then ran me on a treadmill—a stress test. It was normal but showed high cholesterol, borderline diabetes, and elevated blood pressure, which all increased my risk for heart attack. His concise instructions: move more and eat less. I was so far out of shape, I wondered where to start. Then I began thinking about *the bucket*. This simple vessel became my concrete guide to getting fit.

"Picture a plain steel bucket, like the ones you see at the hardware store: gallon-sized with a loop handle. Brand-new buckets are strong and galvanized; they can tolerate an awful lot of abuse and carry anything from milk to hot coals. My grandpa had at least twenty around his farm. The ones he used for milking got washed and dried daily, and those stayed good forever. He used others for watering the horses in their stalls. Over two or three seasons, they'd start to rust. Before they got too leaky, he'd use them for carrying fertilizer, which was fairly corrosive stuff. They'd bang around in the pickup bed as we bounced down farm roads. When a seam would break or a bottom fell out, we'd head to the dump and plink away with his .22 rifle. Then we'd go to town to get some new buckets.

"When I considered my body a steel bucket, good health decisions came easier.

"Over the years, everyone accumulates a few dings. Keep pouring in the hot coals, and you'll get a leaky bucket. Hot coals, in human terms, run the gamut from excess dietary fat to oversized meals. Ensuring the strength of the bucket embraces everything from ample exercise to sufficient sleep. Every meal, every snack, every bite, I thought about what I was putting into the bucket. My diet improved every day. Breakfast bacon became blackberries, and servings got smaller. Within a few weeks, my weight

in nature, and we had to fly to Hawaii. My wife didn't protest.

"Had my grandpa rinsed or even wiped those fertilizer buckets, they might have lasted a little while longer. But buckets were cheap, and we liked shooting. The human reality: buckets always age, and every one of them gets retired eventually. That doesn't mean I shouldn't protect my bucket. I just turned sixty-five and still spend early mornings at the gym or jogging the trail, six days a week. My diet, by some comparisons, is pretty strict. Does this seem like a lot of effort? I don't know anymore, it's just my habit. I do appreciate the intrinsic value of what I'm doing. Researchers estimate the reward is about ten years of life. To me, that has meant spoiling some grandchildren; I've got three so far. It's also led me to a new perspective on medicine. These days, I spend much more time helping prevent problems rather than trying to fix them later.

"Changing our habits is a slow evolution. You both have made excellent progress over the past two months. The example you're setting will place Denise's health on a firm foundation.

"I know we've been focused chiefly on eating right and weight loss. If you're still committed to continue, from here on out, we're going to work on strengthening your buckets. But before starting any exercise program, I recommend a pre-participation exam. Even kids need one before baseball camp.

"You may already have a primary care doctor, but, if not, here's a card for a colleague of mine. Given your youth, it should be minimally invasive, probably no more than a brief exam and EKG. If you were my age, it would be quite a bit more, maybe even a stress test. Next Monday is Veterans Day, and I won't be here. This should give you ample time to get it completed. We'll plan on meeting again in two weeks."

Jack walked Jillian to her car and then returned to his desk. He spent an hour wrapping up a project before he pulled the business card from his shirt pocket and dialed Dr. Williams' friend.

Two minutes later, he had an appointment for the following week. He marked his calendar and reflected back on college: the afternoons spent sweating in the gym and the cool mornings running in the park. He glanced at his feet. "I don't even have decent shoes."

He made a mental note to drop by the running store on Saturday and then dove back into work.

———

At home, Jillian was busy too. She'd already made an appointment with her regular doctor; her annual exam was due next month anyway. Now, she was checking into gym memberships. There were several fitness clubs near their neighborhood, and she believed there was time enough to visit two before school let out. Jillian scooped up her keys and headed back to the garage.

 What are you putting into the bucket?

 How are you strengthening the bucket?

accepted their diaries.

After Jack weighed in and returned to his seat, the doctor faced him squarely. "I got a call from my friend across town. You probably already know, but he's given you the green light to exercise."

Dr. Williams swiveled a bit to face Jillian. "Are you cleared for launch too?"

She nodded brightly.

"I wouldn't have expected anything different for two healthy adults—even patients with heart failure get a prescription for the gym."

The doctor reviewed their diaries then passed them back. "Jillian, I note you've been consistently taking nearly eleven thousand steps every day. That's close to four and a half miles. How do you hit that total?"

She rose slightly in her chair. "I spend about an hour walking laps around our neighborhood every morning."

"That's fantastic. Jack, your daily step count has increased over the past several weeks too."

The doctor hesitated, and Jack disclosed, "I've been trying to walk every day at lunch, about twenty minutes, sometimes more."

Dr. Williams proceeded, "Humans have been walking for around eight million years. It's a graceful, efficient way to move.

Your leg length determines your ideal stride and cadence. Without any special instructions, walkers fall into an economical, natural pace, about three miles per hour. Physicians universally recommend walking for exercise. It's nearly always convenient, requires no special equipment, and has a very, very low injury rate. Walking helps maintain aerobic capacity, bone density, and, as you've both discovered, it burns extra calories, too.

"Some weeks ago, I had mentioned our distant ancestors moved eight to ten miles a day, probably foraging for food. Though it burns calories three times faster than just sitting, walking remains exceptionally frugal. At the natural walking pace, the energy cost to move the human body one mile is rock bottom. For either of you, it's less than a hundred calories. That's probably the only major issue with walking for exercise: it takes a large chunk of time to burn big calories. An ideal exercise program, in the modern sense, has to be balanced against other time commitments, such as family, career, and trivial things like eating and sleeping.

"Jillian, at least for now, you have the ability to commit an hour a day to exercise. I sense, Jack, that you struggle to devote even twenty minutes. Over the past two weeks, you're down barely a pound, swiftly approaching that plateau we discussed. To move beyond it, the next step is literally about stepping, just faster.

"I'm sure you'd join Jillian for her morning walks if work didn't interfere. I'm hoping one day you'll be able to carve out more time for exercise, but, until then, consider substituting duration with intensity, such as running for twenty minutes rather than walking.

"Men walked for about two and a half million years before we added running to our skill set. The advantage of speed comes with a stiff price: it takes far more power to run. The caveman sacrificed this energy in chasing down a wounded animal because it meant steaks for dinner. In modern times, we can use this inef-ficiency to our distinct advantage.

"In your case, Jack, to make better use of your exercise time. When we push ourselves to move faster, the cost to travel a mile

"lunch runners" and had always considered them a little bit silly. As he was reconsidering his opinion, the doctor interrupted, "If nothing else, the extra calories you burned would push you right off this plateau. I'd also point out that's not where the advantages of running end. Because it's a bigger challenge to your heart, car-diovascular fitness improves, and heart attack risk drops. Your muscles demand additional glucose and become more sensitive to insulin, so the risk of diabetes plummets. Of course, you have to be prepared and brown bag it on running days."

Dr. Williams paused, and Jillian offered, "I could help with that."

The doctor nodded to her then looked back at Jack. "I would bet the quality of your lunch would improve. Something else I'd mention is osteoporosis, bone thinning as we age. It's more criti-cal for women, however, moderate running improves bone den-sity in both sexes. Jillian, even though you have time to walk, you may want to consider mixing running days into your routine too.

"How long has it been since either of you ran?" The couple turned toward each other.

"College?" Jillian suggested.

"Yep, it's been that long," Jack agreed.

Dr. Williams resumed, "Then I wouldn't suggest you strap on Nikes and head out for a twenty-minute run. Some weeks after my emergency-room visit, I jumped back in and failed miserably. Though I'd been a decent runner in the army, I hadn't run for at least five years. Army runs were usually a hilly six miles, sometimes even more. My simple plan was three flat miles at the local high school track.

"You've heard about marathoners hitting the wall twenty miles into a run? Legs and lungs fail, and they can't take another step. After the first lap, it felt as if I could reach out and touch the wall. I quit and walked back to the car, utterly dejected.

"Some weeks later, without an ego, I tried again, using a different approach. Rather than risk another public failure, I went to a local hiking trail and tried the run-walk method. At the risk of oversimplification, I began walking at my natural, comfortable pace. There is a speed, somewhere between four and five miles per hour, where it's more humanly comfortable to run. After a minute or two of walking, I stepped up the speed progressively until it felt so awkward I had to break into a jog. It took less than a minute before my lungs told me to stop. Instead of quitting this time, I dropped back to my natural walking pace and caught my breath. Once I recovered, I stepped it up and ran again and then walked some more. Then ran some more. Ten minutes down the trail, I turned around and repeated the process all the way back to the parking lot. This went on for several weeks, though I was walking less and running more. In under a month, I was running the entire twenty minutes.

"I'd forgotten what it takes to become a runner; the price of admission is faithful repetition. Though running is a natural movement, out-of-practice muscles have to remember about working together. Within a few training sessions, however, strides become automatic, and run economy improves. Over a few weeks, there is also a physical transformation in the actual muscle fibers. They assume you'll be running again and learn how to burn fat. In anticipation of your next run, mitochondria, the little power plants of your cells, begin storing energy nearby in little droplets. It takes several minutes to warm up this process. It also takes time to ramp up breathing, heart rate, and oxygen delivery. At the starting line, remember: the first five minutes may actually feel more challenging than the end. This rest-to-run transition shortens to a minute or so with training,

that running might even stimulate joint health. It seems the biggest concern for both novice and experienced runners is over-training, or going too far too soon. Pay close attention to the aches and pains. In the early weeks, you need to be completely recovered between runs. That may mean limiting running to every other day or even every third day.

"With respect to comfortable running, good shoes certainly help. I cringed when I read about Jim Fixx heading out in his old army boots. My suggestion: go to a running-specific store for your first few pairs. Politely excuse yourself and find another store if the sales associate's only question is 'What size do you need?' Before you even try on a pair, they should ask how long you've been running, how far you usually go, and where you do most of your running—track or trail. Only then should they size you up and suggest several different models. The right shoes should balance cushioning against stability but feel comfortable right out of the box. Don't be embarrassed to jog around the parking lot; they should feel good on your feet.

"At the core of human health is exercise. I believe running is the most natural, efficient method we can choose.

"That said, I haven't always been able to run. When I was deployed to the Gulf, my outdoor jogs were abruptly curtailed. I stay indoors on snowy days too. Some of my patients have arthritic conditions that prevent them from running. Other aerobic activities, like swimming, cycling, or rowing, are suitable alternatives. Their benefits are nearly the same as running. Non-running activities have certain other benefits, like no-impact striding on elliptical trainers. The intensity level can be adjusted, and newer machines have built-in heart rate monitors. In any event, the activity you choose should challenge your body with both intensity and duration. My favorite is running, but I sprinkle in others throughout the month for some variety."

That afternoon, Jack phoned Jillian to let her know he'd be a little late. On the way home, he stopped by a small running store. He left thirty minutes later with a pair of trail shoes.

On Tuesday morning, he arrived at work, toting his lunch and a gym bag stuffed with running clothes, new shoes, and a shower kit. He slid everything under his desk and walked to Aaron's office.

Standing in the doorway, Jack thanked him for the referral to Dr. Williams and then moved directly to the point. "Where do you run at lunch?"

Aaron set aside his pen and stood. "I'm glad you're joining us. If you have a moment, we can walk out and I'll show you where the trail starts."

Across town, Jillian had just dropped Denise at school and was trying to decipher Jack's directions to the running store.

 Running burns calories like wildfire.

 Get good shoes, and start slow, slow, slow.

time to change, run, rinse, dress, and, finally, eat. The company course meandered through a city park just a short walk from Alexander Industries. The tree-lined path invoked fond memories of jogging at the university. His pace was slow, but he was walking much less than half the time.

Jack was determined to conquer this two-mile loop within the month. He challenged Jillian's course on Saturday morning, with Denise trailing closely on her bicycle. The effort seemed to lessen as they talked and laughed the whole way. At the end of the second lap, Jack thought or, rather, hoped, this might become a regular weekend adventure. "Much better than cartoons on the couch."

In high school and college, Jillian had only been an occasional athlete. Her track star roommate had tried, on multiple occasions, to coach her into distance running. Dissolving into a panting puddle was her uncomfortable and indelible memory.

Fortunately, the weather was cooperating; mid-November was cool but not yet cold. Best of all, the pace was her own. She structured the run as Dr. Williams described. Twice last week, she walked her first neighborhood loop as usual. Then, stopwatch in hand, she alternated one-minute bursts of running and walking over the entire second loop. The final loop was recovery at her natural pace. She'd been walking sixty minutes daily for nearly three months, so running came far easier than she expected. "Next week," she mused, "I'll just run the middle loop."

———⋄———

Jack stepped off the scale, and Dr. Williams smiled broadly. "Consider the plateau smashed! You're down nearly two pounds from last week."

It was no surprise to Jack. When he'd weighed that morning, his whoop brought Jillian to the bathroom. "Your stellar progress is likely threefold. First, you've expended more energy exercising; running has at least doubled your outlay. Second, the lunches Jillian prepares contain far less calories than typical restaurant fare. Despite monitoring our portions with great caution, we invariably overeat when eating out. Finally, your body is clearly paying attention to what you're doing, tuning appetite to match activity. It's true what they say: dieting improves running, and running improves dieting."

The doctor reached into his drawer and pulled out the measuring tape. "Before we continue, I'd like to check your neck and waist circumferences."

After the doctor measured him several times, Jack returned to his chair quite curious. The doctor revealed no results. "In reality, the core of human work occurs in opposition to gravity. The bones of the body are structurally adapted to counter it. Muscle strength is developed and maintained by working against it. Not long ago, strength was patently necessary for survival. In the past few hundred years, machinery has replaced human brawn and exempted us from a life of physical exertion. Humans have unintentionally acquired patterns of avoiding gravity too: more sitting, less walking, fewer stairs…Without gravity-challenging activities, there is a progressive loss of muscle with aging. Between ages twenty and sixty, muscle mass in men declines by about 40 percent. Women lose nearly 20 percent over the same period, but they start out with significantly less. The medical term for loss of muscle and strength is sarcopenia, essentially, 'poverty of flesh' in Greek. Running is my favorite tool to surgically trim the body back to its foundation. Whether eighteen or

connective tissues develop, enhancing joint stability, especially in the knees and hips. Lifting improves the cholesterol profile and arterial elasticity, and both lower the risk of heart attack. And then there are muscles. Just like running, lifting increases insulin sensitivity and reduces risk for diabetes. Women often worry about bulking up from weight lifting. Even with testosterone, it remains tough enough for men to pack on pounds and pounds of muscle. With training, women gain strong muscles but not big muscles. Though power multiplies, leg measurements actually decrease.

"Cavemen were the first to cross-train; aerobic and strength training are complementary in both form and function. The health benefits overlap and reinforce each other.

"Based on your step count, Jillian, I'm guessing you've already started running. This addition will push your weight loss plateau some weeks, or even months, down the road. Lighter is great, stronger is better still. At any point you choose, I'd suggest trading a few of your walks for a few hours of weight lifting. Muscles require recovery time to repair and grow. A balanced program would alternate days of running with strength training, doing each one two or three days each week.

"I saw Jack's college picture, and I know he's been a gym rat in the past. Have you ever lifted?"

Jillian shook her head.

"Never?"

Another shake.

"Then you have nothing to unlearn. Running is pretty simple. Most everyone can do it for good exercise without any direct coaching. I've found weight lifting to be different, and I wouldn't begin to detail any specific lifting routine. There are innumerable exercises, each with a particular focus. Equipment ranges from one-pound dumbbells and stretchy bands to squat racks and Smith machines.

"It's hardly possible to run three hours a week without seeing notable changes. In contrast, you could spend three hours a day in the gym and make scant progress. While it's possible to begin a program in your basement, my strongest recommendation is to start at a fitness club. The variety and quality of the equipment allows infinite variability as you develop your lifting program. My second bit of advice is to engage a personal trainer to design your initial program with you and then put it into action. They'll start you out light to ensure proper form and confidence in your technique. With hands-on instruction, progress will come much more quickly, though don't expect to see daily changes like you can on a scale. Microscopically, muscle architecture remodeling can be seen in three weeks, but visible changes may take six to seven weeks.

"Jack, I fully understand you are limited by time and not motivation. You landed on a plateau and then broke through it by swapping lunch for a run. Some weeks in the future, you'll find another plateau and have to reconsider your ideal, accounting for all the demands placed on your schedule. You may discover you've picked all the low-hanging fruit.

"From your diary, I calculate you spend about one hundred minutes exercising every week. That's good, however, the surgeon general would suggest we need 150 minutes, minimum, to stay healthy. On the other hand, suppose a man had unlimited time and trained four hours a day. How much fitter could he get? Certainly some, but the benefit curve for exercise flattens quickly at sixty minutes a day. For me, those two numbers place bookends on exercise commitment: two and a half to seven hours per week."

very consistent and reproducible. Jack, you've dropped an honest eighteen pounds. Two and a half months ago, your calculated body fat was a shade over 25 percent—obese by medical standards. Today, you're carrying only 19.1 percent. You've lost more than fifteen pounds of pure fat.

"When you start weight lifting, measuring weight alone won't be enough. Though fat loss is still occurring, it's concealed by muscle growth. Beyond weight, we should measure body fat to assess progress. In ten short weeks, you dropped into the normal-weight category. The athletic range is 10 to 17 percent. You're within striking distance."

———

"Honey," Jillian began as she cleared the table. "I've been thinking about joining a gym. It's going to turn winter soon, and I can't run at the mall. I'm not exactly sure about weight lifting yet. I think I'd be too embarrassed."

Jack offered no resistance. After thinking about it all afternoon, he'd stopped at the local club on his way home. Though he enjoyed running, weight lifting was his choice exercise. He pulled the brochures from his pocket and handed them to Jillian. The hours and rates were already circled.

"If you pack my lunch every day, I believe we can afford it. They even have a kid's area for Denise. I'd get one workout on the weekend, and, it's so close, maybe I could do two mornings or right after work during the week."

He reached out and squeezed her arm gently. "You're gonna look good with Arnold's biceps."

 Challenge gravity with strength training.

 Get a trainer, and start slow, slow, slow.

V V   Though the session at the gym was no longer than her usual run-walk, she was sprinting now to make Monday lunch with Jack.

Over the weekend, she'd moved even more clothes from the spare bedroom. Now the closet was packed.

"This afternoon, I'll do a little cleaning, and you big guys can go."

With a sigh, she grabbed a blouse and slacks to match. Jillian expected to slide into last year's size, but she noted they were a bit snug.

"No way! I've lost more than a pound this week."

Off they came. She was absolutely deflated. In glancing at the tag, she realized her mistake. This pair was her sister's. Forgotten after a visit, they'd hung in the closet for over a year. Jillian looked at the size then laughed out loud. "Now, I know what to wear to the holiday party."

She quickly found her favorite dress. "Old Blue, you're headed to the cleaners."

The doctor handed back their diaries. "Eleven weeks ago, Jack, you presented a concern to me, more about weight but probably an unspoken health worry too.

"Over the same number of weeks, you've embarked on an adventure. You made fundamental changes in both food quantities and choices. I like starting with diet first because it brings on genuine results so quickly. Exercise, however, is what secures success. At first, you added steps and then transitioned to running. While challenging gravity may be optional for work, it's something essential for health, and I see you just started weight lifting.

"In years past, I presented this program in a single visit, and, I believe, my patients found it overwhelming, causing them to balk. Taken step by step, however, everyone has met with success. Not entirely easy, but absolutely doable. Any issues keeping a food diary? Any trouble with counting steps? By now, it's just your habit, like Friday-night lasagna and sundaes were two months ago.

"Making the commitment to change is the biggest hurdle. At home, after my first failed run, I clearly remember changing out of my gym shorts and, again, seeing the big man in the mirror. After years as a soldier, I'd fallen so far and so quickly. Fifty pounds. I'd never known anyone to lose that much weight. It was going to be tough, and I believed fairly well impossible. Wallowing in self-pity, for a moment I simply gave up. It was almost liberating—no calorie counts, no hours of exercise. Eat anything you want. What brought me back from the brink was remembering my grandfather. He was a big-bellied man and showed me how to drive a tractor when I was eight. He died a year later. At the time I was about to give up, my eldest daughter was pregnant with my first grandchild. If I simply surrendered, history would surely repeat itself.

"There is nothing abnormal or shameful about gaining weight. When we overeat and pack on pounds, we're only following our genetic map. Humans are thrifty too. Without predators or competitors forcing us to run, we sit back and relax. These survival instructions were written more than a hundred thousand years ago. Applied today, they have a distinct cost and could shave ten years off your life. A chronic disease like diabetes might make the final twenty a challenge too.

"As a doctor, I understood all this. Understanding is no

the right tools, the executive brain can tame the primitive brain.

"Years later, I still maintain a food diary and exercise log. Both call attention to my bucket—how I'm filling it, how I'm strengthening it. I've also recognized my program is not a zero-sum game. The benefits far outweigh my time investment; there is no paired loss anywhere else in my life. We may measure success by pounds and pant sizes, but the real reward is health.

"This is a graduation day, of sorts. For nearly three months, we've met weekly. There is nothing more to do but continue what you're doing. There are no prohibitions against ice cream or brownies or dining out or a day off now and then. Just keep mindfulness in what you do—protect the bucket.

"I'm happy to see you week to week or month to month. When you're ready, we can even head out for a run."

Jack rose and stood silently for a moment. He extended his hand to the doctor. "Thank you."

 Diet changes bring on results quickly.

 Exercise secures success.

first hustled down this hallway. He tapped on the door and slowly pushed it open.

Dr. Williams face brightened. "How did it go?"

Jack unfurled the T-shirt and displayed it on the doctor's desk. The imprint showed a tennis shoe dancing across a mountaintop. The bold letters underneath read, "Finisher-Mountain States Half-Marathon."

"Congratulations." The doctor folded the shirt and offered it back to Jack.

"No, no. Please keep it. I'll get another. Jillian and I are running one together in three months. Thank you—again."

They shook hands, and Jack exited silently.

Dr. Williams pulled open the bottom drawer and stacked the shirt neatly with the others.

As Jack walked back to his desk, he passed a young man carrying a familiar blue notebook. "You'll do fine," he thought.

Practice Residency Program in Springfield, Missouri.

Dr. Toombs is a 1998 Pisacano Scholar and is board certified in Family Medicine. He serves as the director of the Pain Rehabilitation Center at the Veteran Affairs Medical Center in St. Louis, Missouri.

Dr. Toombs is a veteran of both Desert Storm and Operation Iraqi Freedom, he continues to serve as a physician in the Missouri Army National Guard.

CPSIA information can be obtained
at www.ICGtesting.com
Printed in the USA
LVOW01s0321270416

485504LV00009B/34/P